A POCKET ETYMOLOGY OF MEDICAL TERMS

Printed in Great Britain
ISBN 0-86292-015-9

Published by Bristol Classical Press 1981
Department of Classics
University of Bristol
Wills Memorial Building
Queens Road
Bristol BS8 1RJ

Designed and Printed by Castle Camelot Printers, 131-133 Duckmoor Road, Ashton, Bristol.
Typeset by Quality Phototypesetting Ltd., 26 Oakfield Road, Clifton, Bristol.

PREFACE

Latin and Greek are being studied by fewer and fewer prospective students of medicine, veterinary science, dentistry and allied subjects. Moreover, the etymological basis of the English language is hardly a prominent feature of English courses in schools. For these reasons, medical and paramedical students increasingly find difficulty in understanding medical and scientific terminology and are forced to memorise definitions of individual words, when even a modest acquaintance with etymology would enable them to *work out* the meanings of such words and hence leave their memories free for professional, factual material.

In preparing this book we have attempted to satisfy a need, by providing, not a comprehensive medical dictionary, but a glossary of certain fairly common terms. In addition to – and perhaps more important than – the glossary is the Introduction: this will help readers to understand the construction of the selected words, and enable them to work out the meaning of other words which, for brevity's sake, we have omitted, but which may well be as commonly used as those which are included. We strongly urge all those who use this book to study the Introduction in detail.

Makers of dictionaries are invariably indebted to their predecessors: we have drawn freely on the accumulated wisdom of the standard medical dictionaries and textbooks and the standard dictionaries of English language and etymology. We should also like to single out Walter R. Agard's *Medical Greek and Latin at a Glance* (Paul B. Hoeber, Inc., New York, 1937), since it was after coming across a copy of this book that we decided to produce something comparable.

D.J.A.
R.G.A.B.
Departments of Physiology and Classics & Archaeology
University of Bristol.
1981

CONTENTS

INTRODUCTION

1. The Greek Alphabet and its transliteration

GREEK LETTER	GREEK NAME	TRANSLITERATION IN THIS BOOK
α	alpha	***a***
β	beta	***b***
γ	gamma	***g*** (see note (i) below)
δ	delta	***d***
ε	epsilon	***e*** (short e)
ζ	zeta	***z***
η	eta	***ē*** (long e)
θ	theta	***th***
ι	iota	***i***
κ	kappa	***k***
λ	lambda	***l***
μ	mu	***m***
ν	nu	***n***
ξ	xi	***x***
ο	omicron	***o*** (short o)
π	pi	***p***
ρ	rho	***r*** or ***rh*** (see note (iii) below)
σ (or ς)	sigma	***s***
τ	tau	***t***
υ	upsilon	***u***
φ	phi	***ph***
χ	chi	***ch***
ψ	psi	***ps***
ω	omega	***ō*** (long o)

Notes

(i) Gamma (γ) is transliterated as ***n*** when it immediately precedes kappa (κ) or chi (χ) or xi (ξ) or another gamma. Thus ἐγκεφαλος-*brain* is transliterated as ***enkephalos*** (reflecting the original Greek pronunciation), not ***egkephalos***.

(ii) When ***h*** is found in transliterations from Greek, this represents the so-called 'rough breathing', a mark (') written over a Greek vowel or the second vowel of a diphthong (two vowels in combination) or over a rho (see note (iii) below) to show that it was aspirated: so αἱμα-*blood* is transliterated as ***haima***. Greek words beginning with an *un*aspirated vowel are written with a smooth breathing (') over the vowel. This is not represented in transliteration.

(iii) Rho may sometimes be transliterated as ***r***, sometimes as ***rh***. This corresponds to a distinction in Greek: when rho occurred at the beginning of a word, it was pronounced with an initial aspirate: so e.g. ῥευμα-*a flowing* or *stream* transliterated as ***rheuma***; but when rho occurred anywhere else than at the beginning of a word, it usually lacked the aspirate: so e.g. καρδια-*heart* transliterated as ***kardia***.

N.B. Occasionally ***rh*** will occur in the middle of a transliterated word. This happens when the Greek word is a compound of a prefix plus a second element which begins with a rho. In such cases, if the prefix ends with a vowel, the rho is doubled: e.g. ***diarrhoea***, derived from ***dia-*** (*through*) + ***rhoia*** (*flow, flux*).

(iv) **Accents:** Modern texts of Greek authors are printed with accents: grave (`), acute (´) and circumflex (ˆ). These were invented by a scholar in later antiquity to help foreigners pronounce Greek properly. (It is believed – although the matter is controversial – that these accents indicated the *pitch* at which syllables should be pronounced.) Some systems of transliteration, such as that employed in the *Oxford Dictionary of English Etymology*, retain accents. The main practical advantage of knowing Greek accents is the help which they give one in pronouncing *modern* Greek. For the purposes of this volume it was considered unnecessary to include them. Thus the only textual mark in transliterated Greek here is the *makron* (-), which indicates a long vowel and thus discriminates between epsilon (short e) and eta (long ē) and between omicron (short o) and omega (long ō).

2. Common changes in word-forms from Greek via Latin into English

Some English medical terms are derived from Greek; some from Latin; some from both. When it is a Greek word that lies behind the English one, the form in which that Greek word is borrowed characteristically undergoes a process of 'Latinisation'. The changes concerned (mainly involving vowels) are few, and may be summarised thus:

G.		Eng.	G.	Eng.
ai	→	ae	***haim-***	→ haem-
			anaisth-	→ anaesth-
k	→	c	***kardia***	→ cardi-
			kranion	→ crani-
o	→	u	***karpos***	→ carpus
			oisophagos	→ oesophagus
oi	→	oe	***oidema***	→ oedema
			oisophagos	→ oesophagus
u	→	y	***dus-***	→ dys-
			phusi-	→ physi-

3. Stems

In dictionaries of Greek and Latin, nouns are given in their 'nominative' form, i.e. the form they have when they are acting as the grammatical subject of a sentence. However, the nominative is not always the most useful form to quote if one wishes to understand the classical origin of an English word, since that origin is often seen most clearly if the 'stem' of the noun in question is known. The stem, which may be thought of as the core of the word, acquires various endings in order to distinguish the various roles which the word may play in a sentence. Thus L. ***os****-face* is a nominative; the stem, ***or-***, forms ***oris*** (*of the face*), ***ore*** (*with the face*), etc. It is the stem which gives the clue to such English words as **oral** and **intraoral**. When it seems helpful in this volume to cite the stem as well as the nominative, it is done in this way: ***os/or-***.

Similarly, the form in which Greek and Latin verbs are given in dictionaries (the first-person singular present indicative active, corresponding to the translation *I walk, I go,* etc.) and the other commonly-cited form (the 'infinitive', corresponding to the translation *to walk, to go,* etc.) are not always the most illuminating from the point of view of English etymology. The Latin verb meaning *I lead*, ***duco***, with infinitive ***ducere***, can throw direct etymological light on such English words as *adduce* or *reduce*; but, in order to perceive the derivation of words like *conductor* or *induction*, one needs to be aware that ***duco/ducere*** changes to ***duct-*** in certain circumstances. In cases where neither the 'dictionary' form nor the infinitive is as useful for etymological purposes as some other form of the verb, that other form is usually given in this volume as well. Thus **retroflexion** is glossed as ***retro*** (*backwards*) + L. ***flectere/flex-*** (*bend*): ***flectere*** is the infinitive; ***flex-*** is related to a grammatical form known as the 'supine'. (The supine is often the form of a Latin verb from which English derivatives come. Thus L. ***manere***, *to remain*, has a supine ***mansum***, whence Eng. *mansion*; L. ***videre***, *to see*, has supine ***visum***, whence *vision, visible,* etc.)

4. Common prefixes in medical terms

This section is intended to serve as no more than a rough guide. In particular, it must not be assumed that a given prefix will always form compounds which are parallel in meaning.

(i) This is especially true in relation to Greek prepositions like **kata-, dia-, meta-** and **para-,** which had several distinct meanings. English derivatives of these prepositions often preserve the distinctions. An instance is the role of **meta-** in **metabolism** and **metacarpal**. In **metabolism**, it connotes *change* (cf. **metamorphosis**); in **metacarpal** its sense might be described as spatial: *after, beyond – that which comes after the carpus* (*wrist*).

(ii) More subtle, but no less important, are the kinds of variation in meaning associated with compound words beginning with e.g. **endo-, post-** and **supra-**. Here a core meaning (*within, behind, above*) persists, but the relation between prefix and second element is sometimes 'prepositional' (**endocarditis** = (*inflammation*) *within the heart*) and sometimes 'adjectival' (**endoderm** = *inner* (*germinal layer*).

The list which follows provides, where possible, one biological example (introduced 'so') and, for comparison, one non-biological word with the same prefix (introduced 'cf.'). For abbreviations used in this list, in the list of suffixes which follows, and in the glossary, see p. 15.

a- (or, before vowel or *h,* **an-**) G. prefix (i) *absence of* (ii) *deficiency of*
so (i) **aphasia:** ***a-*** + G. ***phas-,*** *speech* = *speechlessness*
cf. **asymmetrical** = *not symmetrical*
so (ii) **anaemia:** ***an-*** + G. ***haima,*** *blood* = *deficiency of blood*
N.B. Beware of confusion with ***ana-****, q.v.*

ab- L. prep. *away from*
so **abductor:** ***ab-*** + L. ***ducere/duct-,*** *lead* = *that which leads away*
cf. **abnormal** = *that which deviates from what is normal*

ad- L. prep. *to, towards, near*
so **adrenal:** ***ad-*** + L. ***renes,*** *kidneys* = *near the kidneys*
cf. **adhere** (L. ***haerere***, *to stick*) = *stick to*
N.B. In a number of *ad-* compounds the *d* alters under the influence of the next letter to form a double consonant: e.g. **afferent** = *leading towards*

ambi- L. prep. (found only in compound words) *both*
so **ambidextrous:** ***ambi-*** + L. ***dextr-,*** *right hand* = *able to use both hands as if they were one's right hand* (*i.e. equally well*)
cf. **ambiguous** = *of double meaning*

ana- G. prep. *up, again, back*
so **anatomy:** ***ana-*** + G. ***tom-,*** *cut* = *cutting up, separation into constituent parts*
cf. **anagram** (G. ***graphein,*** *to write*) = *that which results when a word is broken up and written again* (*differently*)
N.B. There is a danger of confusing ***ana-*** with ***an-*** compounds; the two groups must just be memorised as there is no convenient way of distinguishing them by their form

ante- L. prep. and advb. *before*
so **antenatal:** ***ante-*** + L. **natalis**, *connected with, relating to, birth = before birth*
cf. **antecedent** (L. ***cedere***, *to go*) = *that which goes before (something else)*
N.B. Beware of confusion with ***anti-***, *q.v.*

anti- G. prep. *against*
so **antibiotic:** ***anti-*** + G. ***bios***, *life = a substance which inhibits life processes*
cf. **antithesis** (G. ***thesis***, *placing*) = *that which is set against or opposed to*
N.B. Beware of confusion with ***ante-***, *q.v.*

bi- L. prefix (related to L. advb. **bis**, *twice*) *double*
so **bilaminar:** ***bi-*** + L. ***lamina***, *a thin plate or layer = double-layered*
cf. **bicentennial** = *the two-hundredth anniversary*

cata- G. prep. (***kata***) with several connotations, the two most relevant being (i) *down*
(ii) *thoroughly, completely*
so (i) **catarrh:** ***kata-*** + G. ***rhein,*** *to flow = a discharge which flows down*
cf. **catastrophe** (G. ***strephein/stroph-,*** *to turn*) = *a violent down-turn, overthrow*
so (ii) **catalepsy:** ***kata-*** + G. ***lēpsis***, *seizure = seizure, trance* (see Glossary entry)
cf. **catalogue** = *complete list, complete record*

circum- L. prep. *around*
so **circumoral:** ***circum-*** + L. ***os/or-,*** *mouth,* = *around the mouth*
cf. **circumnavigate** = *sail round*

con- (or **com-** when immediately before a 'labial' consonant, e.g. *b, m, p*) L. prefix (found only in compound words) from L. prep. ***cum***, *with*
so **commensal:** ***com-*** + L. ***mensa***, *table = sharing a table; an organism which lives in another with benefit to itself and no disadvantage to the host*
cf. **compassion** (L. ***pati/pass-***, *to suffer*) = *suffering with*

contra- L. prep and advb. *against, opposite*
so **contralateral:** ***contra-*** + L. ***latus/later-***, *side* = *on the opposite side*
cf. **contradict** (L. ***dicere/dict-***, *to say*) = *speak against, oppose in speech*

de- L. prep. *down from, away from*
so **denervate:** ***de-*** + L. ***nervus***, *sinew, bowstring, nerve* = *deprive of nerves*
cf. **decapitate** (L. ***caput/capit-***, *head*) = *to remove the head*

di- prefix (related to G. advb. ***dis***, *twice*) *double*
so **digastric:** ***di-*** + G. ***gastēr/gastr-***, *belly* = *having two bellies* (applied to a muscle with that structure)
cf. **dilemma** = *a problem involving a choice between two equally unfavourable alternatives*

dia- G. prep. (i) involves idea of motion *through* something
(ii) implies *thoroughness* or *completeness*
so (i) **diarrhoea:** ***dia-*** + G. ***rhoia***, *flow, flux* = *fluid faeces which flow through*
cf. **diaphanous** (G. ***phainein/phan-***, *to show*) = (*something*) *that allows light to pass through it*
so (ii) **diagnosis:** ***dia-*** + G. ***gnōsis***, *knowledge* = *thorough knowledge and identification of a medical condition*

dys- G. prefix (found only in compound G. words) implies *difficulty, being wrong* or *unfavourable*
so **dysentery:** ***dys-*** + G. ***enteron***, *guts* = *bad guts*, i.e. *inflammation of large intestine*
N.B. The ancient grammarian Didymos was nicknamed ***Chalkenteros***, *Brass Guts*, because of his amazing capacity for hard work

e- (or **ex-**) L. prep. *out of, from*
so **exsanguinate:** ***ex-*** + L. ***sanguis/sanguin-***, *blood* = *to make bloodless*
cf. **emit** (L. ***mittere***, *to send*) = *send out*

ec- (or **ex-**) G. prep. *out of, from*
so **eczema:** ***ek-*** + G. ***zema***, *boiling* = *a 'boiling-out' of the skin* (inflammation)
cf. **ecstasy** (G. ***stasis***, *state, condition*) = *a state of being outside one's normal wits*

ecto- from G. prep and advb. ***ektos***, *outside*
so **ectoderm:** ***ekto-*** + G. ***derma***, *skin* = *outer skin*

en- (or **em-** when immediately before a 'labial' consonant, e.g. *b, m, p, ph*) G. prep. *in*
so **emphysema:** ***em-*** + G. ***phusa-***, *blow up, puff up* = *distension by air or gas*
cf. **embalm** = *place into balm* (i.e. *spice*)

endo- from G. advb. ***endon*** (*within*) (i) *inside* (ii) *inner*
so (i) **endocarditis:** ***endo-*** + G. ***kardia***, *heart* = *inflammation within the heart*
(ii) **endoderm:** ***endo-*** + G. ***derma***, *skin* = *inner layer*

epi- G. prep. *upon*
so **epidermis:** ***epi-*** + G. ***derma***, *skin* = *that which is upon the skin; outer layer of the skin*
cf. **epitaph** (G. ***taphos***, *tomb*) = *that which is (written) upon a tomb*

extra- L. prep. and advb. *outside*
so **extracranial:** ***extra-*** + G. ***kranion***, *skull* = *outside the cranium* (*skull*)
cf. **extraterrestrial** (L. ***terra***, *earth*) = *that which is placed, or which happens, outside the Earth*

hemi- G. prefix (found only in compound G. words) *half*
so **hemiplegia:** ***hemi-*** + G. ***plēgē***, *stroke, blow* = *stroke to, paralysis of, one side of the body*
cf. **hemisphere** (G. ***sphaira***, *ball*) = *a half-sphere*

homo- (also **hom(o)eo-**) G. adj. *the same*
so **homolateral:** ***homo-*** + L. ***latus/later-***, *side* =

situated on the same side
cf. **homosexual** = *having an interest in the same sex*

hyper- G. prep. *above, too much, too great*
so **hypertrophy:** ***hyper-*** + G. ***trophē***, *nourishment* = *excessive growth (of an organ)*
cf. **hypermarket** = *an extremely (? excessively) large market*
N.B. Beware of confusion with ***hypo-***, *q.v.*

hypo- G. prep. (i) *below, beneath* (ii) *deficient*
so (i) **hypodermic:** ***hypo-*** + G. ***derma***, *skin* = *below the skin*
cf. **hypothesis** (G. ***thesis***, *placing*) = *a principle set down as a basis for arguing*
so (ii) **hypothermia:** ***hypo-*** + G. ***thermos***, *hot* = *deficient (below normal) body temperature*
N.B. Beware of confusion with **hyper-**, *q.v.*

inter- L. prep. *between*
so **intercostal:** ***inter-*** + L. ***costa***, *rib* = *between the ribs*
cf. **international** = *taking place between nations*

intra- L. prep. and advb. *within*
so **intracellular:** ***intra-*** + L. ***cellula***, *a small storeroom* (diminutive of ***cella***, *chamber* or *storeroom*) = *within a cell*
cf. **intramural** (L. ***murus***, *wall*) = *that which is within walls*

intro- L. advb. *within*
so **introversion:** ***intro-*** + L. ***vertere/vers-***, *to turn* = *a turning inwards* (see Glossary entry)
cf. **introduce** (L. ***ducere***, *to lead*) = *to lead into*

meta- G. prep. conveys notion of (i) *change* (ii) *sequence (after)*
so (i) **metastasis:** ***meta-*** + G. ***stasis***, *state, condition, position* = *transference (of e.g. diseased cells) from one part to another*
cf. **metamorphosis** (G. ***morph-***, *form*,

shape) = *change of form*
so (ii) **metacarpal** = *the part of the hand situated after the carpus* (*wrist*)
cf. **Metaphysics** = *the work of Aristotle which came after his* Physics

ortho- G. adj. *upright, straight, correct*
so **orthopaedic:** ***ortho-*** + G. ***pais/paid-*** (also diminutive form ***paidion***) *child* = *connected with the correction of deformities* (literally *'in children'*, but in people generally)
cf. **orthodox** (G. ***doxa***, *opinion*) = *holding 'correct'* – e.g. *generally accepted – views*

para- G. prep. (with a wide range of senses in Greek: *from, at, beside, beyond, to the side of,* etc.); the two main (related) meanings which **para-** has in English compounds are (i) *by the side*
(ii) *amiss, wrong*
so (i) **parathyroid:** ***para-*** + G. ***thureos***, *an oblong shield* (***thura***, the ultimate derivation, means *door*); whence *thyroid, shield-shaped* = *alongside, adjacent to, the thyroid gland*
cf. **parallel** (G. ***allēlos***, *one another*) = (*lines*) *lying alongside one another*
so (ii) **paraesthesia:** ***par(a)-*** + G. ***aisthēs-***, *sensation* = *abnormal sensation*
cf. **paradox** (G. ***doxa***, *opinion*) = *an opinion contrary to prevailing opinions* or *an apparently self-contradictory opinion*

peri- G. prep. *around*
so **pericardium:** ***peri-*** + G. ***kardia***, *heart* = *that* (membranous sac) *which surrounds the heart*
cf. **periscope** (G. ***skopein***, *to look*) = *device for looking around*
N.B. the *different* relation between **peri-** and the second element in some other compounds, e.g. **peritoneum**, where G. ***tonos*** comes from ***teinein***, *to stretch*. The whole word means *that* (*membrane*) *which is stretched around* (*and encloses*) *the contents of the abdominal cavity.*

post- L. prep. and advb. (i) *behind* (ii) *after*
so (i) **post-ocular:** ***post-*** + L. **oculus**, *eye = behind the eye*
so (ii) **postnatal:** ***post-*** + L. ***natalis***, *relating to birth = after birth*
cf. **Post-impressionism** = *an artistic movement which came after Impressionism*

pre- from L. prep. and advb. ***prae***, *before, in front of*
so **precordium,** ***pre-*** + L. ***cor/cordis***, *heart = the region in front of the heart* (and stomach)
cf. **precede** (L. ***cedere***, *to go*) = *go before, in front of*

pro- G. prep. *beforehand*
so **prognosis:** ***pro-*** + G. ***gnōsis***, *knowledge = anticipation* (*of probable course of a disease*)
cf. **prologue** (G. ***logos***, *word, speech*) = *preliminary or introductory speech*

retro- L. advb. *backwards*
so **retroflexion:** ***retro-*** + L. ***flectere/flex-***, *to bend = being bent backwards*
cf. **retroactive** = *acting in a backward direction*

sub- L. prep. *under*
so **subcranial:** ***sub-*** + G. ***kranion***, *skull = beneath the skull*
cf. **subterranean** (L. ***terra***, *earth*) = *beneath the earth* (*surface*)

supra- L. prep & advb. *above*
so **suprarenal:** ***supra-*** + L. ***renes***, *kidneys = situated above the kidneys*

syn- (or **sym-** when immediately before a 'labial' consonant, e.g. *b, m, p, ph*) G. prep. *with, together*
so **symphysis:** ***sym-*** + G. ***phusis***, *natural growth = a growing-together or union* (*e.g. of two bones*)
cf. **symphony** (G. ***phōnē***, *voice*) = *harmony of sound*

trans- L. prep. *across*
so **transfusion:** ***trans-*** + L. ***fundere/fus-***, *to*

pour = process of conveying a fluid (e.g. blood) from one vessel to another
cf. **transport** (L. ***portare***, *to carry*) = verb *to convey from one place to another* or noun. *the means of such conveyance*

5. *Common suffixes in medical terms*

-cyte used in the formation of names of cell-types (G. ***kutos***, *something hollow, a vessel, a container*; hence the use of the word for a biological receptacle, the cell)
so **histiocyte:** G. ***histion*** (diminutive of ***histos***) *web, something woven, tissue,* + ***-cyte*** *= a connective tissue cell*

-gen (also **-genesis, -genic, -genous**) derived from G. suffix ***-genēs***, which is in turn related to G. vbs. ***gignesthai***, *to become* and ***gennan***, *to produce, to bring forth.* The suffixes therefore give to compounds in which they occur the sense *producing* or *production*
so **lactogenic:** L. ***lac/lact-***, *milk,* + ***-genic*** *= stimulating the production of milk*

-ia a very common G. suffix used to form abstract nouns; unlike e.g. **-cyte, -gen** or **-logy** it has no special 'meaning'. In Eng. it is often used to denote *a condition of*
so **hypothermia:** G. ***hupo-***, *below,* + G. ***thermos***, *hot* + ***-ia*** *= a condition of being below normal body temperature*

-itis a suffix which is widely employed in forming names of diseases which involve inflammation. The logic of choosing this particular ending is apparently as follows: a group of adjectives in G. end in ***-itēs*** when agreeing with a masculine noun, but in ***-itis*** when agreeing with a feminine noun. Now, the G. word for a *disease* is ***nosos***, which is feminine. Thus the G. for *disease of the kidney* is ***nephritis nosos***; or ***nephritis*** for short.

The usage has in Eng. been particularised to connote *inflammation* rather than just *disease* so **lymphangitis:** L. ***lympha***, *water,* + G. ***angos*** (also ***angeion***, *vessel, receptacle*) = *inflammation of a lymph node*

-lysis in compound words means *breaking down* (from G. ***lusis***, *loosening*)
so **haemolysis:** G. ***haima***, *blood,* + ***-lysis*** = *the dissolution of red corpuscles*
cf. **electrolysis** = *chemical decomposition by electricity*

-oid derived from G. noun ***eidos***, *form,* and connoting *formed like*
so **arachnoid:** G. ***arachnē***, *a spider,* + ***-oid*** = *web-like* (applied to one of the membranes covering the brain)
cf. **anthropoid** (G. ***anthrōpos***, *human being*) = *human in form*

-(o)logy from G. ***logos***, *word, speech, reason*; in Eng. compounds, *study, science*
so **cardiology:** G. ***kardia***, heart, + ***-logy*** = *the study or science of the heart*
cf. **sociology** (L. ***socius***, *colleague, fellow*) = *the study or science of society* (*one's fellow men*)

-oma many G. nouns end thus. As with **-ia**, the suffix has no 'meaning'; in Eng. medical usage **-oma** is used to form names of tumours or other morbid growths
so **angioma:** G. ***angos*** (also ***angeion***, *vessel, receptacle*) + **-oma** = *a tumour involving blood or lymph vessels*

-osis common G. ending for nouns involving the notion of *process* or *condition*. When used to form Eng. medical terms it often indicates a pathological condition
so **necrosis:** G. ***nekrōsis***, *mortification* (from ***nekros***, *corpse* + ***-osis***) = *death of a tissue or organ*

-pathy G. ***pathos*** means *experience, feeling*, i.e. *that which happens to one,* or *that which one suffers.* In Eng. compounds **-pathy** may mean simply *feeling* (as in **sympathy**, *feeling with*), but in medical words it often connotes *disease*

so **neuropathy:** G. ***neuron****, sinew, tendon,* later *nerve,* + ***-pathy*** = *disease in nerves*

GLOSSARY

Notes to users of glossary

1. An asterisk ***before** a word in the glossary means that it begins with a prefix whose usage is described in Section 4 of the Introduction above.
2. An asterisk **after*** a word in the glossary means that it ends with a suffix whose usage is described in Section 5 of the Introduction above.
3. *q.v.* (L. ***quod vide****, which see*) means that the word just mentioned should be looked up at its alphabetical place in the glossary.
4. When a glossary entry for word X ends 'cf. Y' (cf. is an abbreviation for L. ***confer****, compare, contrast*), the reader should **always** look up Y in the glossary in order to see the relationship between X and Y.

* * *

A

***a-** (or, before a vowel or *h*, **an-**): G. negating prefix indicating *absence* or *deficiency*.

***ab-:** L. prefix meaning *away from*.

abdomen: L. noun, stem ***abdomin-***, meaning *lower part of the belly* (the region between the diaphragm and the pelvic floor).

abduct:** (ab-***, *q.v.*, + L. ***ducere/duct-***, *to lead*) *to draw away* (from the midline of the body).

aberrant:** (ab-***, *q.v.*, + L. ***errare***, *to wander*) *deviating from the normal or usual course.*

ablate:** (ab-***, *q.v.*, + L: ***lat-***, *carried* – derived from L. ***ferre***, *to carry*) *to remove or take away.*

acapnia*:** (a-***, *q.v.*, + G. ***kapnos***, *smoke*, + ***-ia***, *q.v.*) *absence of carbon dioxide* (cf. **hypo-** and **hypercapnia**)

achalasia*:** (a-***, *q.v.*, + G. ***chalan***, *to relax*, + ***-ia***, *q.v.*) *failure* (of a muscle sphincter) *to relax.*

achlorhydria*:** (a-***, *q.v.*, + G. ***chlōros***, *pale green*, + G. ***hudōr***, *water*, + ***-ia***, *q.v.*) *absence of hydrochloric acid in the gastric juice* (chlorine, of which hydrochloric acid is a compound, is a greenish-yellow gas).

achondroplasia*:** (a-***, *q.v.*, + G. ***chondros***, *lump, gristle, cartilage*, + G. ***plassein***, *to form, to mould, to shape*, + ***-ia***, *q.v.*) *disordered growth of bones which normally develop from cartilage.*

achromatic:** (a-***, *q.v.*, + G. ***chrōma***, *colour*) *colourless, not staining* (in histology); *a lens in which chromatic aberration is corrected* (in optics).

achylia*:** (a-***, *q.v.*, + G. ***chulos***, *juice*, + ***-ia***, *q.v.*) *lack of digestive juice* (usually gastric or pancreatic juice).

acidaemia*: (L. ***acidus***, *sour, acid*, + ***haem-***, *q.v.*, + ***-ia***, *q.v.*) *abnormally acid blood*, i.e. lower than normal blood pH.

acinus (pl. **acini**): L. word meaning *berry*, esp. *grape*, hence *grape-like component of a gland* (often one of many, as in a bunch of grapes).

acromegaly: (G. ***akros***, *topmost, outermost, extreme*, + G. ***megas/megal-***, *large, great*) *continued* or *recommencement of growth in adult life* (characterized by elongation of the extremities and the lower jaw).

acupuncture: (L. ***acus***, *needle*, + L. ***pungere/punct-***, *to prick*) *penetration of the skin with needles.*

***ad-:** L. prefix meaning *to, towards, near.*

adduct:** (ad-***, *q.v.*, + L. ***ducere/duct-***, *to lead*) *to move towards* (the midline of the body).

adenopathy*: (G. ***adēn***, *gland*, + ***-pathy***, *q.v.*) *disease of a gland.*

adiadochokinesis:** (a-***, *q.v.*, + G. ***diadochos***, *in succession, taking over from one another*, + G. ***kinēsis***, *movement*) *clumsiness, inability to arrest one movement and change to another.*

adipose: (L. ***adeps/adip-***, *fat*) *fatty.*

adrenal:** (ad-***, *q.v.*, + L. ***renes***, *kidneys*) *near the kidneys* (the adrenal glands are sometimes called **suprarenal**, i.e. *above the kidneys*).

adrenergic:** (ad-***, *q.v.*, + L. ***renes***, *kidneys*, + G. ***ergon***, *work, function*) *functioning by the production of adrenaline* (a secretion of the adrenal glands).

aerobic: (G. ***aēr***, *air*, + G. ***bios***, *life*) *using air* (oxygen) *for living.*

aerophagy: (G. ***aēr***, *air*, + G. ***phagein***, *to eat*) *the swallowing of air.*

aesthesia*: (G. ***aesthēs-***, *sensation, feeling*, + ***-ia***, *q.v.*) *sensibility, feeling.*

aetiology*: (G. ***aitia***, *cause*, + ***-logy***, *q.v.*) *the study or science of causation* (generally applied to diseases).

afferent:** (ad-***, *q.v.*, + L. ***ferre***, *to carry*) *carrying centrally* (applied to nerves and nerve impulses) or *towards an organ* (applied to blood vessels).

agglutination: (L. verb ***agglutinare***, *to glue, to stick to*) *sticking to* (generally applied to the clumping together of red corpuscles or other cells or particles).

agglutinogen*: (L. ***agglutinare***, *to glue, to stick to*, + ***-gen***, *q.v.*) *an agent which brings about agglutination.*

albinism: (L. ***albus***, *white*) *whiteness* (due to congenital absence of pigment).

algesia*: (G. ***algos***, *pain*, + ***-ia***, *q.v.*) *the condition of pain.*

alimentary: (L. ***alimentum***, *nourishment*, from L. ***alere***, *to feed, to nourish*) generally used as adjective with *canal*, meaning *the digestive tract.*

alveolus (pl. **alveoli**): (L. noun meaning *a small cavity*) *a rounded space in bone* (alveolar bone), *in a gland* or *in the lungs.*

alymphocytosis*:** (a-***, *q.v.*, + L. ***lympha***, *water*, + G. ***kutos***, *something hollow, a vessel*, or *a container* (hence its use for *a cell*), + ***-osis***, *q.v.*) *absence of cells which are formed in the lymphatic system* (lymphocytes) – sometimes implies very few, not complete absence.

***ambi-:** L. prefix meaning *both.*

ambidextrous:** (ambi-***, *q.v.*, + L. ***dexter***, *right*, i.e. that which is on the right-hand side, therefore by common experience *skilful, handy*) *able to use both hands with equal skill.*

amenorrhoea:** (a-***, *q.v.*, + G. ***mēn***, *month*, + G. ***rhoia***, *flow, flux*) *absence of menstrual* (monthly) *flow*.

amnesia*:** (a-***, *q.v.*, + G. ***mnē***, root of several G. words connoting *memory* and *remembering*, + ***-ia***, *q.v.*) *failure of the memory*.

amorphous:** (a-***, *q.v.*, + G. ***morph-***, *form, shape*) *formless*; (in chemistry) *non-crystalline*.

amylase: (G. ***amulon***, *starch*, + ***-ase***, a suffix – with no Greek or Latin pedigree – indicating *an enzyme* which acts on the substance indicated in the first part of the word; so **proteinase, carbohydrase**, etc.) *an enzyme which acts upon starch and starch-like compounds*.

amyloid*: (G. ***amulon***, *starch*, + ***-oid***, *q.v.*) *starch-like*.

***ana-:** G. prefix meaning *up, back, again*.

anabolism:** (ana-***, *q.v.*, + G. ***bol-***, from ***ballein***, *to throw*) *building up* (cf. **catabolism** and **metabolism**).

anaemia*:** (a-/an-***, *q.v.*, + ***haem-***, *q.v.*, + ***-ia***, *q.v.*) literally *deficiency of blood*; *inadequate oxygen-carrying capacity of the blood* (owing to deficiency of red corpuscles and/or functional haemoglobin).

anaerobe:** (a-/an-***, *q.v.*, + ***aerob(ic)***, *q.v.*) *a micro-organism which lives without air* (oxygen).

anaesthesia*:** (a-/an-***, *q.v.*, + ***aesthesia***, *q.v.*) *absence of sensation* (cf: **hyper-** and **paraesthesia**).

anaplasia*:** (ana-***, *q.v.*, + G. ***plassein***, *to form, to mould, to shape*, + ***-ia***, *q.v.*) *reversal from a more to a less differentiated form* (***ana-*** here in sense of *backwards*).

anastomosis*:** (G. noun meaning *opening, outlet*, derived from ***ana-, *up*, + G. ***stoma***, *mouth*, whence ***anastomō***, *I provide with a mouth*, i.e. *open up*) *communication between blood vessels; joining-up between structures*.

anatomy:** (ana-***, *q.v.*, + G. ***tom-***, *cut*) literally *cutting up* (the first technique employed in the science of form and structure).

androgen*: (G. ***anēr/andr-***, *man* (as opposed to woman; man as opposed to beast is G. ***anthrōpos***), + ***-gen***, *q.v.*)

producing male characteristics (term frequently applied to male hormones).

androgynism: (G. ***anēr/andr-***, man, + G. ***gunē,*** *woman*) *hermaphroditism* (*q.v.*).

aneurysm: (G. noun ***aneurusmos,*** *dilatation*, from G. ***eurus,*** *wide*) *dilatation of a blood vessel* (usually an artery).

angina: (L. noun meaning *the quinsy*, related to G. ***anchein,*** *to throttle*) *a condition characterized by a feeling of tightness, constriction* or *suffocation.*

angiocardiogram: (G. ***angos***, also ***angeion,*** *vessel, receptacle,* + G. ***kardia,*** *heart,* + common Eng. suffix ***-gram***, derived from G. ***gramma,*** *that which is written down*) *an X-ray record of the appearance of the heart and great vessels* (obtained after injecting radio-opaque material into the circulation).

(N.B. Compounds ending in ***-gram*** often have companion compounds ending in ***-graph***, an Eng. suffix which means *the instrument used for writing or drawing*; thus **telegram**, **telegraph**)

angioma* (pl. **angiomata**): (G. ***angos***, also ***angeion,*** *vessel, receptacle,* + ***-oma,*** *q.v.*) *a tumour involving blood or lymph vessels.*

anhydrous:** (a-***, *q.v.*, + G. ***hudōr,*** *water*) *absence of water* (generally applied to chemical compounds).

ankylosis*: (G. ***ankulos,*** *crooked, curved,* hence ***ankulē,*** *the 'bend' of a joint,* + ***-osis,*** *q.v.*) literally *joint pathology*, but applied to *immobility of a joint.*

anorexia*:** (a-/an,*** *q.v.*, + G. ***orexis,*** *yearning, longing,* + ***-ia,*** *q.v.*) *no appetite.*

anoxaemia*:** (a-/an,*** *q.v.*, + G. ***oxus,*** *sharp* – oxygen was so called because it was thought to give rise to acid (sharp) compounds – + ***haem-,*** *q.v.*, + ***-ia,*** *q.v.*) literally *no oxygen in the blood*; but in common (and inexact) usage *less than normal blood oxygen.*

anoxia*:** (a-/an,*** *q.v.*, + G. ***oxus*** – cf. **anoxaemia** – + ***-ia,*** *q.v.*) *no oxygen* (often erroneously used instead of the correct term **hypoxia** (*q.v.*) to denote *less than normal oxygen level*).

antagonist: (***anti-***, *q.v.*, + G. ***agōnistēs***, *a competitor, a rival*) *a muscle, nerve, endocrine gland or drug which opposes the action of another.*

***ante-:** L. prefix meaning *before.*

antenatal:** (ante-***, *q.v.*, + L. ***natalis***, *relating to birth*) *before birth.*

***anti-** G. prefix meaning *against.*

antibiotic:** (anti-***, *q.v.*, + G. ***bios***, *life*) *a substance which inhibits life processes.*

antibody:** (anti-***, *q.v.*, + Eng. ***body***) literally *an against substance* (found in body fluids and a component of the bodily defence system).

antidromic:** (anti-***, *q.v.*, + G. ***dromos***, *race course*, or *the act of running*) *contrary to the usual direction.*

antigen*:** (anti-***, *q.v.*, + ***-gen***, *q.v.*) *a substance which evokes a defence reaction* (specifically the formation of antibodies).

antitoxic:** (anti-***, *q.v.*, + G. ***toxikos***, *connected with a bow and arrow*; then, when applied to a drug, *for smearing arrows with* – hence, by implication, *poisonous*) *acting against a poisonous substance* (toxin).

antrum (pl. **antra**): (L. noun meaning *cave*) *a cavity in bone*; also *part of the stomach.*

anuria*:** (a-***, *q.v.*, + G. ***ouron***, *urine*, + ***-ia***, *q.v.*) *absence of urine.*

aphagia*:** (a-***, *q.v.*, + G. ***phagein***, *to eat*, + ***-ia***, *q.v.*) *inability to swallow* (cf. **dysphagia**).

aphasia*:** (a-***, *q.v.*, + G. ***phas-***, *speech*, + ***-ia***, *q.v.*) *inability to articulate words* and/or *to understand spoken words.*

aplasia*:** (a-***, *q.v.*, + G. ***plassein***, *to form, to mould, to shape*, + ***-ia***, *q.v.*) *failure to develop.*

apnoea:** (a-***, *q.v.*, + G. ***pnoia***, a form of ***pnoē***, *breath*) *absence of breathing* (cf. **dys-, eu-** and **hyperpnoea**).

apocrine: (G. verb ***apokrinein***, *to separate*) *a gland in which part of the secretory cell separates off with the secretory fluid.*

arachnoid*: (G. ***arachnē***, *a spider*, + ***-oid***, *q.v.*) *web-like* (applied to one of the membranes covering the brain).

arrhythmia: (***a-***, *q.v.*, + G. ***rhuthmos***, *measured time, proportion, regularity*, + ***-ia***, *q.v.*) *lack of rhythm; irregularity.*

arthritis*: (G. ***arthron***, *joint*, + ***-itis***, *q.v.*) *inflammation of a joint.*

asphyxia: (***a-***, *q.v.*, + G. ***sphuxis***, *beating, throbbing pulsation*, + ***-ia***, *q.v.*) literally *no beating*, by common usage *no breathing* (and generally applied to suffocation involving no gas exchange and therefore accumulation of carbon dioxide and absence of oxygen).

asthenia*: (G. ***asthenēs***, *weak*, + ***-ia***, *q.v.*) *lack of strength* (an 'asthenic' person is characteristically tall and slender).

asynergia: (***a-***, *q.v.*, + G. ***sunergia***, *co-operative activity, working with*, + ***-ia***, *q.v.*) *lack of co-ordination of activity* (in muscle groups which normally work together).

ataxia: (G. noun meaning *disorder*, formed from ***a-***, *q.v.*, + G. ***taxis***, *order, arrangement*, + ***-ia***, *q.v.*) *disordered arrangement* (usually referring to unco-ordinated movements).

atonia: (***a-***, *q.v.*, + G. ***tonos***, *that which is stretched*, hence *strain, tension*, + ***-ia***, *q.v.*) *lack of tension* (cf. **hypotonia**).

atrium (pl. **atria**): (L. noun meaning *hall, entrance room*) *entrance* or *first part of the heart* (through which the blood flows).

atrophy**: (G. ***atrophia, *lack of nourishment*, formed from ***a-***, *q.v.*, + ***trophē***, *nourishment*) *wasting of a part* (often but not always due to local nutritional deficiency).

auscultation: (L. verb ***auscultare***, *to listen to*) *examination by listening.*

autolysis*: (G. ***autos***, *self*, + ***-lysis***, *q.v.*) *breakdown of cells or organs by self-originating enzymes.*

autonomic: (G. ***autos***, *self*, + G. ***nomos***, *law, habit, rule*) *self-governing, independent* (applied to part of the nervous system not under direct voluntary control).

avascular**: (a-***, *q.v.*, + L. ***vasculum***, *small vessel*, diminutive of ***vas***, vessel) *without blood vessels.*

B

bacillaemia*: (L. ***bacillus***, *q.v.*, + ***haem-***, *q.v.*, + ***-ia***, *q.v.*) *bacilli in the blood.*

bacillus (pl. **bacilli**): (L. noun meaning *a small rod or staff*) *a rod-shaped micro-organism.*

bacteriocidal: (G. ***baktērion***, *a small rod or staff*, + ***-cide***, Eng. suffix derived from L. ***-cida***, *one who kills*) *destroying bacteria.*

bacteriolysis*: (G. ***baktērion***, *a small rod or staff*, + ***-lysis***, *q.v.*) *dissolution of bacteria.*

bacteriophage: (G. ***baktērion***, *a small rod or staff*, + G. ***phagein***, *to eat*) *substance which has bacteriolytic action* (see **bacteriolysis**).

bacteriostasis: (G. ***baktērion***, *a small rod or staff*, + G. ***stasis***, *a stoppage, a standstill*) *cessation of bacterial growth.*

bacterium (pl. **bacteria**): (G. ***baktērion***, *a small rod or staff*) *unicellular micro-organism.*

ballistocardiograph: (L. ***ballista***, *machine for hurling projectiles*, from G. ***ballein***, *to throw*, + G. ***kardia***, *heart*, + ***-graph*** – see **angiocardiogram**) *an apparatus for recording recoil movements of the body in relation to the heart beat.*

baroreceptor: (G. ***baros***, *a load, a weight*, + L. ***recept-***, from ***recipere***, *to receive*) *pressure receptor.*

***bi-:** L. prefix meaning *double.*

bilaminar:** (bi-***, *q.v.*, + L. ***lamina***, *a thin plate or layer*) *double-layered.*

bilateral:** (bi-***, *q.v.*, + L. ***latus/later-***, *side*) *on two sides.*

bioenergetics: (G. ***bios***, *life*, + G. ***energeia***, *activity, working, operation*) *energy turnover in living organisms.*

biopsy: (G. ***bios***, *life*, + G. ***opsis***, *sight, vision*) *tissue removed from the living organism for examination.*

bradycardia*: (G. ***bradus***, *slow, sluggish*, + G. ***kardia***, *heart*, + ***-ia***, *q.v.*) *slow heart-beat.*

bronchiectasis: (G. ***bronchos***, *windpipe*, + G. ***ektasis***, *a stretching out, extension*) *dilatation of the bronchi.*

buccolingual: (L. ***bucca***, *the cheek*, + L. ***lingua***, *the tongue*) *associated with or near to the cheek and tongue.*

C

cachexia*: (G. ***kakos***, *bad, evil*, + G. ***hexis***, *state, condition*, + ***-ia***, *q.v.*) *severe debilitation* (frequently associated with advanced malignant disease).

calorimetry: (L. ***calor***, *heat*, + G. ***metron***, *measure*) *heat measurement.*

capillary: (L. ***capillus***, *a hair*) *a minute, hairlike vessel* (in the cardiovascular and lymphatic systems).

cardiology*: (G. ***kardia***, *heart*, + ***-logy***, *q.v.*) *the study or science of the heart.*

***cata-:** G. prefix meaning *down, thoroughly* or *completely.*

catabolism:** (cata-***, *q.v.*, + G. ***bol-***, from ***ballein***, *to throw*) *breakdown of molecules* (cf. **anabolism** and **metabolism**).

catalepsy:** (cata-***, *q.v.*, + G. ***lēpsis***, *seizure*) *sustained posture of limbs or body in positions in which they are passively placed* (often associated with hysteria or hypnosis).

catalyst:** (cata-***, *q.v.*, + G. ***luein***, *to undo*) *substance which facilitates a chemical reaction.*

catarrh:** (cata-***, *q.v.*, + G. ***rhein***, *to flow*) *discharge which 'flows down'* (associated with inflammation of a mucous membrane).

caudal: (L. ***cauda***, *tail*) *relating to tail end or lower part of the body.*

causalgia*: (G. ***kausos***, *fever*, related to ***kaiein***, *to burn*, + G. ***algos***, *pain*, + ***-ia***, *q.v.*) *burning pain.*

centrifugal: (L. ***centrum***, = G. ***kentron***, *centre*, originally *the sharp point of a pair of compasses*, hence *the centre of a circle so produced*, + L. ***fugere***, *to flee*) *moving from the centre.*

centripetal: (L. ***centrum*** – see **centrifugal** – + L. ***petere***, *to seek*) *moving towards the centre.*

cephalic: (G. ***kephalē***, *the head*) *relating to the head* (sometimes to the brain).

cervical: (L. ***cervix/cervic-***, *the neck*) *relating to the neck of the body or structures in the neck or to the narrower portion of an organ.*

chalone: See **hormone**.

cheilitis*: (G. ***cheilos***, *a lip*, + ***-itis***, *q.v.*) *inflammation of the lip.*

cholecystokinin: (G. ***cholē***, *gall, bile*, + G. ***kustis***, *bladder*, + G. ***kinein***, *to move*) *a substance which causes contraction of the gall bladder.*

chromatolysis*: (G. ***chrōma/chrōmat-***, *colour*, + ***-lysis***, *q.v.*) *loss of colour* (generally loss of staining reaction of the substance chromatin in the nucleus of degenerating cells).

chronotropic: (G. ***chronos***, *time*, + G. ***trop-***, from ***trepein***, *to turn*) *affecting rate* (applied to heart rate) (cf. **inotropic**).

chylomicron (pl. **chylomicra**): (G. ***chulos***, *juice*, + G. ***mikros***, *small*) *small particle(s)* (of fat) *absorbed into the blood from the gut.*

circadian: (L. ***circa***, *around*, + L. ***dies***, *day*) *a daily cycle of events.*

***circum-:** L. prefix meaning *around.*

circumoral:** (circum-***, *q.v.*, + L. ***os/or-***, *mouth*) *around the mouth.*

circumvallate:** (L. verb ***circumvallare, *to surround with a wall*, from ***circum-***, *q.v.*, + ***vallum***, *an earthen wall, a rampart*) *surrounded by an elevation or wall.*

commensal:** (con-***, *q.v.*, + L. ***mensa***, *a table*) *an organism which lives in another* (with benefit to itself and no disadvantage to the host).

commissure: (L. noun ***commissura***, *a joining together*) *a connecting pathway* (generally across the midline in the central nervous system).

***con- (com-):** L. prefix meaning *with*.

contagious: L. ***contagio***, *contact, infection*, from ***con-***, *q.v.*, + ***tangere***, *to touch*) *spreading by contact.*

***contra-:** L. prefix meaning *against, opposite.*

contralateral.** (contra-**, q.v.,* + L. ***latus/later-**, side*) *on the opposite side.*

corticofugal: (L. ***cortex/cortic-**, rind, bark,* + L. ***fugere**, to flee*) *moving from the outer layer of an organ* (such as the brain, kidney or suprarenal gland).

corticotrophin: (L. ***cortex/cortic-**, rind, bark,* + G. ***trophē**, nourishment*) literally *nourishing the cortex* (applied to a hormone which stimulates the suprarenal cortex to secrete).

cryosurgery: (G. ***kruos**, icy cold,* + Eng. ***surgery***) *surgery performed with the aid of extreme cold.*

cryptorchism: (G. ***kruptein**, to hide,* + G. ***orchis**, testicle*) *failure of the testicles to descend into the scrotum.*

cyanosis*: (G. ***kuanos**, dark blue,* + ***-osis**, q.v.*) *blue colour of the tissues* (usually resulting from the presence of deoxyhaemoglobin, a blue pigment, in the blood).

-cyte*: suffix used in names of types of cell; from G. ***kutos**, something hollow, a vessel, a container*; hence the use of the word for a biological receptacle, the cell.

cytolysis*: (G. ***kutos**, something hollow* (see ***-cyte***), + ***-lysis**, q.v.*) *cell breakdown.*

D

***de-:** L. prefix meaning *down from, away from.*

decerebrate:** (de-**, q.v.,* + L. ***cerebrum**, the brain*) *to remove the brain* (specifically, to cut the connection between the upper and lower regions of the brain).

decussation: (L. verb ***decussare**, to divide in the form of the letter X*) *a crossing-over* (in the shape of the letter X).

defibrinate:** (de-**, q.v.,* + ***fibrin***, from L. ***fibra**, a fibre*) *to remove fibrin from blood.*

deglutition: (L. ***deglutio**, I swallow down*) *the process of swallowing.*

dendrite: (G. ***dendron**, a tree*) *a cell process like the branches of a tree.*

denervate:** (de-**, q.v.,* + L. ***nervus**, sinew, bowstring, nerve*) *to deprive of nerves.*

dermatology*: (G. ***derma/dermat-**, skin,* + ***-logy**, q.v.*) *the study or science of skin* (normal and abnormal).

dermatome: (G. ***derma/dermat-**, skin,* + G. ***tom-**, cut*) *a clearly demarked area of skin* (supplied by a single spinal nerve).

desmosome: (G. ***desmos**, bond, ligature,* + G. ***sōma**, body*) *structural link between cell bodies.*

***dia-:** G. prefix connoting *through,* or *thoroughness.*

diagnosis:** (dia-**, q.v.,* + G. ***gnōsis**, knowledge*) *thorough knowledge and identification of a medical condition.*

dialysis*:** (dia-**. q.v.,* + ***-lysis**, q.v.*) *passage of water and dissolved crystalloid substances through a membrane*, and, by implication, *the retention of large molecules.*

diarrhoea:** (dia-**, q.v.,* + G. ***rhoia**, flow, flux*) *flowing of fluid faeces.*

diastole: (G. noun meaning *a drawing apart*) *relaxation of muscle* (specifically heart muscle).

digastric:** (di-**, q.v.,* + G. ***gastēr/gastr-**, belly*) *having two bellies* (applied to a muscle with that structure).

diplopia*: (G. ***diplous**, double,* + G. ***ōps**, eye,* + ***-ia**, q.v.*) *double vision.*

diurnal: (L. ***diurnus**, daily*, from L. ***dies**, day*) *referring to a daily event or one occurring during the day.*

dorsal: (L. ***dorsum**, the back*) *relating to the back or posterior part of the body.*

dorsiflexion: (L. ***dorsum**, the back,* + L. ***flectere/flex-**, to bend*) *bending backwards or posteriorly.*

***dys-:** G. prefix implying *difficulty, being wrong* or *unfavourable.*

dysarthria*:** (dys-**, q.v.,* + G. ***arthron**, a joint,* + ***-ia**, q.v.*) literally *badly-jointed,* applied particularly to badly-articulated (L. ***articulus**, a small joint*) speech; hence, *impaired speech, difficulty in articulating words.*

dysentery:** (dys-***, *q.v.*, + G. ***enteron***, *guts*) *inflammation of large intestine.*

dyskinesia*:** (dys-***, *q.v.*, + G. ***kinein***, *to move*, + ***-ia***, *q.v.*) *impairment of movement.*

dyslexia*:** (dys-***, *q.v.*, + G. ***lexis***, *speech, diction, style, phrase*, + ***-ia***, *q.v.*) *difficulty with reading* (perhaps *complete inability to read*).

dysmetria*:** (dys-***, *q.v.*, + G. ***metron***, *measure*, + ***-ia***, *q.v.*) *difficulty in judging distance* (when performing movements).

dysphagia*:** (dys-***, *q.v.*, + G. ***phagein***, *to eat*, + ***-ia***, *q.v.*) *difficulty in swallowing* (cf. **aphagia**).

dysplasia*:** (dys-***, *q.v.*, + G. ***plassein***, *to form, to mould, to shape*, + ***-ia***, *q.v.*) *abnormal tissue formation* (cf. **hyperplasia**).

dyspnoea:** (dys-***, *q.v.*, + G. ***pnoia***, a form of ***pnoē***, *breath*) *difficulty, discomfort and distress in breathing* (cf. **a-**, **eu-**, and **hyperpnoea**).

dystrophy:** (dys-***, *q.v.*, + G. ***trophē***, *nourishment*) *degenerative changes of an organ or tissue* (associated with local nutritional defects).

E

***e-** (or **ex-**): L. prefix meaning *out of, from.*

***ec-** (or **ex-**): G. prefix meaning *out of, from.*

ecbolic:** (ec-***, *q.v.*, + G. ***bol-***, from ***ballein***, *to throw*) *expelling* (applied to the secretory function of gland cells or the expulsive action of the uterus or the foetus).

ecto-:** from ***ektos, G. prefix meaning *outside.*

ectoderm:** (ecto-***, *q.v.*, + G. ***derma***, *skin*) literally, *outer skin* (applied to outer embryonic germinal layer).

ectopic:** (ec-***, *q.v.*, + G. ***topos***, *place*) *in an abnormal place.*

eczema:** (ec-***, *q.v.*, + G. ***zema***, *boiling*) *inflammation* (boiling-out) *of the skin.*

electrocardiogram: (G. ***ēlektron***, originally *amber,* from which static electricity can be generated – in this compound *to do with electrical activity* –, + G. ***kardia****, heart,* + ***-gram*** – see **angiocardiogram**) *a record of the electrical activity of the heart.*

embolus** (pl. **emboli**): (en-/em-****, q.v.,* + G. ***bol-***, from ***ballein****, to throw*) *a detached part of a blood clot or a collection of cells or air which obstructs a blood vessel.*

emetic: (G. ***emetikos****, promoting vomit*) *that which brings about vomiting* (emesis).

emphysema:** (en-/em-****, q.v.,* + G. ***phusa-****, blow up, puff up*) *distension by air or gas.*

***en-** (or **em-**): G. prefix meaning *in.*

endo-:** from ***endon, G. prefix meaning *inside.*

endocarditis*:** (endo-*** *q.v.,* + G. ***kardia****, heart,* + ***-itis****, q.v.*) *inflammation, within the heart, of the lining membrane* (the endocardium).

endocrine:** (endo-****, q.v.,* + G. ***krinein****, to separate*) *relating to internal secretion* (secretion involves separation of fluid from the blood).

endoderm:** (endo-****, q.v.,* + G. ***derma****, skin*) *inner* (embryonic germinal) *layer* (cf. **ectoderm**).

endogenous (***endo-****, q.v.,* + ***-genous****; q.v.*) *formed or produced within* (the body or a cell).

endometrium** (pl. **-tria**): (endo-****, q.v.,* + G. ***mētra****, womb*) *the inner lining of the uterus.*

endoneurium** (pl. **-neuria**): (endo-****, q.v.,* + G. ***neuron****, sinew, tendon,* later *nerve*) *the internal tissue immediately surrounding the nerve axons within a bundle.*

enzyme:** (en-****, q.v.,* + G. ***zumē****, ferment* or *leaven*) originally *a substance which facilitates fermentation*; now applied to *biological catalysts.*

***epi-:** G. prefix meaning *upon.*

epidemic: (G. ***epidēmios****, among a people*, (of a disease) *prevalent*) *a widespread infectious disease.*

epidermis:** (epi-**, q.v.,* + G. ***derma**, skin*) *outer layer of the skin.*

ergometer: (G. ***ergon**, work,* + G. ***metron**, measure*) *an apparatus for measuring* (muscular) *work.*

erythema (pl. **-meta**): (G. noun meaning *redness of the skin*) *redness of the skin.*

erythrocyte*: (G. ***eruthros**, red,* + ***-cyte**, q.v.*) *a red cell* (corpuscle).

erythropoiesis: (G. ***eruthros**, red,* + G. ***poiēsis**, making*) *the formation of red corpuscles.*

eupnoea: (G. ***eu**, well,* + G. ***pnoia***, a form of ***pnoē**, breath*) *normal breathing* (cf. **a-, dys-** and **hyperpnoea**).

exfoliation:** (e-/ex-**, q.v.,* + L. ***folium**, leaf*) *loss of flakes* (leaves); e.g. loss of surface layers (of skin).

exophthalmos:** (ec-/ex-**, q.v.,* + G. ***ophthalmos**, eye*) *protruding eye.*

exostosis (pl. **exostoses**): (***ec-/ex-**, q.v.,* + G. ***osteon**, bone,* + ***-osis**, q.v.*) *bone growth projecting beyond normal surface.*

exsanguinate:** (e-/ex-**, q.v.,* + L. ***sanguis/sanguin-**, blood*) *to make bloodless.*

exteroceptor: (L. ***exterus**, that which is on the outside,* + L. ***-cept-***, from ***capere**, to take*) *receptor for stimuli originating outside the body.*

***extra-:** L. prefix meaning *outside.*

extracranial:** (extra-**, q.v.,* + G. ***kranion***, skull) *outside the cranium* (skull).

extravascular:** (extra-**, q.v.,* + L. ***vasculum**, small vessel*, diminutive of ***vas**, vessel*) *outside a vessel.*

F

febrile: (L. ***febris**, fever*) *like or associated with a fever.*

fenestrated: (L. ***fenestra**, window*) *with openings* (a fenestrated membrane has gaps in it).

filiform: (L. ***filum**, thread* + L. ***forma**, form, shape*) *threadlike.*

foramen (pl. **foramina**): (L. noun meaning *opening* or *aperture*) *a hole.*

fungiform: (L. ***fungus***, *mushroom*, + L. ***forma***, *form, shape*) *mushroom-shaped.*

G

galactose: (G. ***gala/galakt-***, *milk*) *a monosaccharide* (derived by hydrolysis of lactose, the sugar in milk).

ganglion (pl. **ganglia**): (G. ***ganglion***, *tumour*) *a collection of cells and supporting tissue* (in the nervous system), or *a fluid swelling.*

gastric: (G. ***gastēr/gastr-***, *belly*) *relating to the stomach.*

gastroenterology*: (G. ***gastēr/gastr-***, *belly*, + G. ***enteron***, *gut*, + ***-logy***, *q.v.*) *the study or science of the stomach and intestines.*

-gen*, -genesis*, -genic*, -genous*: suffixes derived from G. suffix ***-genēs***, which is in turn related to G. verbs ***gignesthai***, *to become*, and ***gennan***, *to produce, to bring forth*; the suffixes therefore give to compounds in which they occur the sense *producing* or *production.*

geratology*: (G. ***gēras***, *old age*, + ***-logy***, *q.v.*) *the study or science of old age.*

geriatric: (G. ***gēras***, *old age*, + G. ***iatros***, *doctor, one who heals*) *relating to treatment of old age.*

gluconeogenesis*: (G. ***glukus***, *sweet*, + G. ***neos***, *new*, + ***-genesis***, *q.v.*, *production, coming-into-being*) *glucose formation from non-carbohydrate* (and therefore new) *sources.*

glycaemia*: (G. ***glukus***, *sweet*, + ***haem-***, *q.v.*, + ***-ia***, *q.v.*) *glucose in the blood.*

glycogenesis*: (G. ***glukus***, *sweet*, + ***-genesis***, *q.v.*, *production, coming-into-being*) glycogen formation (strictly speaking the word ought to be **glycogengenesis**).

glycogenolysis*: (***glycogen***, from G. ***glukus***, *sweet*, + ***-gen***, *q.v.*; + ***lysis***, *q.v.*) *breakdown of glycogen* (a sugar-producing substance).

gynaecology* (G. ***gunē/gunaik-***, *woman*, + ***logy***, *q.v.*) *the study or science of normal and abnormal function in females.*

H

haem- (or **haemat-**): (G. ***haima/haimat-***, *blood*) used in compound words connected with *blood*.

haemangioma* (pl. **-omata**): (***haem-***, *q.v.*, + G. ***angos***, also ***angeion***, *vessel, receptacle*, + ***-oma***, *q.v.*) *a growth originating in blood vessels.*

haematemesis: (***haem(at)-***, *q.v.*, + G. ***emein***, *to vomit*) *the vomiting of blood* (cf. **haemoptysis**).

haematocrit: (***haem(at)-***, *q.v.*, + G. ***krit-***, from ***krinein***, *to separate*) *an instrument in which red cells and plasma are separated centrifugally* (in order to determine their relative proportions).

haematology*: (***haem(at)-***, *q.v.*, + ***-logy***, *q.v.*) *the study or science of the blood.*

haematoma* (pl. **-omata**): (***haem(at)-***, *q.v.*, + ***-oma***, *q.v.*) *a swelling containing blood.*

haemodynamics: (***haem-*** *q.v.*, + G. ***dunamis***, *power, force*) *the physical principles governing blood pressure and flow.*

haemolysis*: (***haem-***, *q.v.*, + ***-lysis***, *q.v.*) *the dissolution of red corpuscles.*

haemopoiesis: (***haem-***, *q.v.*, + G. ***poiēsis***, *making*) *blood formation.*

haemoptysis: (***haem-***, *q.v.*, + G. ***ptuein***, *to spit*) *the spitting of blood* (from haemorrhage in the respiratory tract) (cf. **haematemesis**).

haemorrhage: (***haem-***, *q.v.*, + G. ***rhag-***, from ***rhēgnunai***, *to break*) *blood loss.*

haemostasis: (***haem-***, *q.v.*, + G. ***stasis***, *stoppage, standstill*) *the arrest of blood flow.*

***hemi-:** G. prefix meaning *half*.

hemianopia*:** (hemi-***, *q.v.*, + ***a-/an-***. *q.v.*, + G. ***ōps***, *eye*, + ***-ia***, *q.v.*) *blindness of half of the visual field.*

hemiatrophy:** (hemi-**, q.v.,* + ***atrophy**, q.v.*) *one-sided atrophy.*

hemiplegia*:** (hemi-**, q.v.,* + G. ***plēgē**, stroke, blow,* + ***-ia**, q.v.*) *paralysis of one side of the body.*

hermaphroditism: (G. ***Hermaphroditos***, a mythological character combining attributes of both sexes) *a mixture of male and female characteristics.*

heterogeneous: (G. ***heteros**, different,* + G. ***genos**, sort, kind*) *differing, not originating from the same kind or population.*

hidrosis*: (G. ***hidrōs**, sweat,* + ***-osis**, q.v.*) *excessive,* or *abnormal sweating.*

histiocyte*: (G. ***histion***, diminutive of ***histos**, web, something woven, tissue,* + ***-cyte**, q.v.*) *a connective tissue cell* (general term; cf. **osteocyte**).

histology*: (G. ***histos**, web, something woven, tissue* + ***-logy**, q.v.*) *the study or science of tissues.*

***homo-/hom(o)eo-:** G. prefix meaning *the same.*

hom(o)eostasis:** (hom(o)eo-**, q.v.,* + G. ***stasis**, stoppage, standstill, state, condition*) *equilibrium, constancy* (of which a stable body temperature, blood sugar level, etc., are examples).

hom(o)eothermal:** (hom(o)eo-**, q.v.,* + G. ***thermos**, hot*) of constant temperature (generally applied to warm-blooded animals) (cf. **poikilothermal**).

homolateral:** (homo-**, q.v.,* + L. ***latus/later-**, side*) *on the same side.*

homologous:** (homo-**, q.v.,* + G. ***logos***, here *rationale, rational basis*) *identical structure or type.*

homunculus: (L. ***homunculus**, little man,* diminutive of ***homo***, *human being*) *little man* (a proportional representation of the body in the motor and sensory areas of the cerebral cortex).

hormone: (G. verb ***horman**, to incite, to set in motion*) literally *a stimulating substance* (applied to chemicals liberated by endocrine glands which excite other cells; substances which *inhibit* other cells were originally called **chalones** – G. ***chalan**, to relax* – but **hormone** is now common usage for *all* endocrine secretions, whether stimulating or inhibiting).

humoral: (L. ***(h)umor***, *fluid*) *relating to body fluids,* (commonly excluding blood).

hydrocele: (G. ***hudōr***, *water,* + G. ***kēlē***, *swelling*) *a swelling containing a water* (serous) *fluid.*

hydrolysis*: (G. ***hudōr***, *water,* + ***-lysis***, *q.v.*) *chemical dissolution /breakdown, involving preliminary combination with water.*

hygrometer: (G. ***hugros***, *moist,* + G. ***metron***, *measure*) *an instrument for the measurement of the moisture content* (of air).

***hyper-:** G. prefix meaning *above, too much, too great.*

hyperaemia*:** (hyper-***, *q.v.*, + ***haem-***, *q.v.*, + ***-ia***, *q.v.*) *greater than normal blood flow.*

hyperaesthesia*:** (hyper-***, *q.v.*, + ***aesthesia***, *q.v.*) *raised sensitivity* (cf. **an-** and **paraesthesia**).

hypercapnia*:** (hyper-***, *q.v.*, + G. ***kapnos***, *smoke,* + ***-ia***, *q.v.*) *greater than normal carbon dioxide level* (cf. **a-** and **hypocapnia**).

hyperglycaemia*:** (hyper-***, *q.v.*, + G. ***glukus***, *sweet,* + ***haem-***, *q.v.*, + ***-ia***, *q.v.*) *higher than normal blood sugar level* (cf. **hypoglycaemia**).

hypermetropia*:** (hyper-***, *q.v.*, + G. ***metron***, *measure,* + G. ***ōps***, *eye,* + ***-ia***, *q.v.*) *long-sightedness* (light rays 'overshoot' the retina to focus beyond it).

hyperplasia*:** (hyper-***, *q.v.*, + G. ***plassein***, *to form, to mould, to shape,* + ***-ia***, *q.v.*) *increased number of cells in a tissue or organ causing an increase in size* (cf. **hypertrophy** and **dysplasia**).

hyperpnoea:** (hyper-***, *q.v.*, + G. ***pnoia***, a form of ***pnoē***, *breath*) *overbreathing* (cf. **a-**, **dys-** and **eupnoea**).

hyperpyrexia*:** (hyper-***, *q.v.*, + ***pyrexia***, *q.v.*) *very high body temperature.*

hypertrophy:** (hyper-***, *q.v.*, + G. ***trophē***, *nourishment*) *increased size of a tissue or organ due to enlargement of its constituent cells* (cf. **hyperplasia**).

***hypo-:** G. prefix meaning *below, beneath, deficient.*

hypocapnia*:** (hypo-***, *q.v.*, + G. **kapnos**, *smoke*, + **ia**, *q.v.*) *lower than normal level of carbon dioxide* (cf. **a-** and **hypercapnia**.)

hypodermic:** (hypo-***, *q.v.*, + G. **derma**, *skin*) *beneath the skin.*

hypoglycaemia*:** (hypo-***, *q.v.*, + G. **glukus**, *sweet*, + **haem-**, *q.v.*, + **-ia**, *q.v.*) *lower than normal blood sugar level* (cf. **hyperglycaemia**).

hypothermia*:** (hypo-***, *q.v.*, + G. **thermos**, *hot*, + **ia**, *q.v.*) *below normal body temperature.*

hypotonia*:** (hypo-***, *q.v.*, + G. **tonos**, *that which is stretched*, hence *strain, tension*, + **ia**, *q.v.*) *less than normal tension* (cf. **atonia**).

hypoxia*:** (hypo-***, *q.v.*, + G. **oxus**, *sharp* – cf. **anoxaemia** – , + **-ia**, *q.v.*) *less than normal oxygen* (cf. **anoxia**).

hysterectomy: (G. **hustera**, *womb*, + G. **ektom-**, *cutting out*) *removal of the uterus.*

I

-ia*: suffix used in the formation of names of abnormal or pathological conditions.

iatric: (G. **iatros**, *doctor, one who heals*) *relating to a physician or the practice of medicine.*

iatrogenic*: (G. **iatros**, *doctor, one who heals*, + **genic**, *q.v.*) *referring to disorders arising during, and in some way attributable to, treatment of a disease* (literally *produced by a doctor* – contrast **icterogenic**).

icterogenic*: (G. **ikteros**, *jaundice*, + **-genic**, *q.v.*) *producing jaundice* (contrast the function of ***-genic*** here with its function in **iatrogenic**).

idiopathy*: (G. **idios**, *one's own, relating to oneself*, + **-pathy**, *q.v.*) *disease or disorder of spontaneous origin* (as far as we know, within the existing limitations of science).

idiosyncrasy: (G. **idios**, *one's own, relating to onself*, + G. **sunkrasis**, *mixing together*) *an individual characteristic.*

imbibition: (L. **imbibere**, *to drink*) *taking up fluid.*

immunology* (L. ***immunis***, *exempt from*, + **-*logy***, *q.v.*) *the study or science of protective mechanisms.*

inanition: (L. ***inanis***, *empty*) *lack of food* (to the extent of starvation).

incontinence: (***in***-, negating prefix (cf. **incapable**), + L. ***continere***, *to retain, to contain*) *inability to retain* (faeces or urine).

ingestion: (L. ***ingerere/ingest-***, *to bring in*) *the taking in of food* (a preliminary to digestion).

inotropic: (G. ***is/in-***, pl. ***ines***, *fibres*, + G. ***trop-***, from ***trepein***, *to turn*) *affecting the ability of muscle fibres to contract* (cf. **chronotropic**).

insulin: (L. ***insula***, *island*) *a hormone produced by islets* (small islands of Langerhans in the pancreas).

***inter-:** L. prefix meaning *between.*

intercostal:** (inter-***, *q.v.*, + L. ***costa***, *rib*) *between the ribs.*

***intra-:** L. prefix meaning *within.*

intramural:** (intra-***, *q.v.*, + L. ***murus***, *wall*) *within the wall* (used in referring to structures within the wall of a hollow structure or organ such as a blood vessel or the gut).

***intro-:** L. prefix meaning *within.*

introversion:** (intro-***, *q.v.*, + L. ***vertere/vert-***, *to turn*) *turning in of the cut end of a tube*, or *an inward-turning mental attitude.*

ipsilateral: (L. ***ipse***, *self, oneself, himself*, etc., + L. ***latus/later-***, *side*) *on the same side.*

ischaemia*: (G. ***ischein***, *to hold back*, + ***haem-***, *q.v.*, + ***-ia***, *q.v.*) *lack of* or *absence of blood.*

isometric: (G. ***isos***, *equal*, + G. ***metron***, *measure*) *of equal* or *unchanging length.*

isotonic: (G. ***isos***, *equal*, + G. ***tonos***, *that which is stretched*; hence *strain, tension*) (also applied to solutions which, when cells are suspended in them, cause no change in the intracellular tension).

-itis*: suffix used in the formation of names of diseases involving inflammation.

J

juxtaglomerular: (L. ***juxta,*** *nearby,* + L. ***glomus/glomer-*** *a ball of yarn*) *near the glomerulus* (a knot or ball of capillaries in the kidney).

K

karyolysis*: (G. ***karuon,*** *nut,* + ***-lysis,*** *q.v.*) *disintegration of the cell nucleus* (a nut-like structure).

kinaesthesia*: (G. ***kinein,*** *to move,* + ***aesthesia,*** *q.v.*) *combined sensations of weight, position and movement.*

kinesiology*: (G. ***kinesis,*** *movement,* from ***kinein,*** *to move,* + ***-ology,*** *q.v.*) *the study or science of movement.*

L

lactogenic* (L. ***lac/lact-,*** *milk,* + ***-genic,*** *q.v.*) *stimulating the production of milk.*

laevorotatory: (L. ***laevus,*** *left,* + L. ***rotare,*** *to turn*) *rotating* (the plane of polarised light) *to the left.*

laparotomy: (G. ***lapara, flank,*** + G. ***tom-,*** *cut*) *an incision through the flank* (abdominal wall).

leucocyte*: (G. ***leukos,*** *white,* + ***-cyte,*** *q.v.*) *white* (blood) *cell.*

leucopenia: (G. ***leukos,*** *white,* + G. ***penia,*** *poverty*) *low concentration of white cells in the blood.*

leucoplakia*: (G. ***leukos,*** *white,* + G. ***plax/plak-,*** *plain, flat land,* + ***-ia,*** *q.v.*) *inflammatory condition characterized by white patches* (seen on the tongue, oral or genital mucosa).

leukaemia*: (G. ***leukos,*** *white,* + ***haem-,*** *q.v.,* + ***-ia,*** *q.v.*) *a pathological condition of which an increase in the number of white cells in the blood is one feature.*

lipoid*: (G. ***lipos***, *animal fat, lard,* + ***-oid***, *q.v.*) *fat-like substances, insoluble in water.*

lipolytic: (G. ***lipos***, *animal fat,* + ***-lytic***, derived from G. ***lusis***, *loosening, dissolution*) *fat-splitting.*

lithotomy: (G. ***lithos***, *stone,* + G. ***tom-***, *cut*) *an incision* (into the bladder) *to remove a stone.*

-logy*: suffix from G. ***logos***, *word, speech, reason*; in Eng. compounds, *study, science.*

lymphagogue: (L. ***lympha***, *water,* + G. ***agōgos***, *leading*) *a substance which stimulates lymph flow.*

lymphangitis* (L. ***lympha***, *water,* + G. ***angos***, also ***angeion***, *vessel, receptacle,* + ***itis***, *q.v.*) *inflammation of a lymph node.*

lymphocyte*: (L. ***lympha***, *water,* + ***-cyte***, *q.v.*) *white corpuscle produced in the lymphatic system.*

lymphopoiesis: (L. ***lympha***, *water,* + G. ***poiēsis***, *making*) *the formation of* **lymphocytes**.

-lysis*: suffix meaning *breaking down,* from G. ***lusis***, *loosening,* which is in turn from ***luein***, *to loosen.*

lysozyme: (G. ***luein***, *to loosen,* + G. ***zumē***, *ferment* or *leaven*) *a substance in various secretions and in plants, capable of breaking down bacterial cells.*

M

macroscopy: (G. ***makros***, *large,* + G. ***skopein***, *to view*) *looking at with the naked eye* ('large-viewing' as opposed to – with a microscope – 'small-viewing').

malnutrition: (L. ***malus***, *bad,* + L. ***nutrio***, *nourish*) *defective nourishment.*

megaloblast: (G. ***megas/megal-***, *large,* + G. ***blastos***, *shoot, germ*) *large immature cell.*

melanophore: (G. ***melas/melan-***, *black,* + G. ***phoros***, *bearing, carrying*) *a cell which contains the dark pigment melanin.*

meninges: (G. pl. of noun ***mēninx***, *membrane*) *the membranes* (of the brain and spinal cord).

menopause: (G. ***mēn***, *month*, + G. ***pauein***, *to stop*) *cessation of menstrual* (monthly) *flow*.

menstrual: (L. ***menstrualis***, *monthly*, from ***mensis***, *month*) *relating to monthly flow*.

mesencephalon: (G. ***mesos***, *middle*, G. ***enkephalon***, *brain*) *the midbrain*.

mesoderm: (G. ***mesos***, *middle*, + G. ***derma***, *skin*) *middle embryonic germinal layer*.

***meta-:** G. prefix connoting *change* or *sequence*.

metabolism:** (G. ***metabolē, *change*, from ***meta-***, *q.v.*, + ***bol-***, from ***ballein***, *to throw*) *all the chemical changes in the body* (including **anabolism**, *q.v.*, and **catabolism**, *q.v.*).

metacarpal:** (meta-***, *q.v.*, + G. ***karpos***, *wrist*) *relating to the part of the hand situated after or beyond the carpus* (wrist).

metamorphosis*:** (meta-***, *q.v.*, + G. ***morph-***, *form, shape*, + ***-osis***, *q.v.*) literally *change in form* (with special significance in biology and pathology).

metaplasia*:** (meta-***, *q.v.*, + G. ***plassein***, *to form, to mould, to shape*, + ***-ia***, *q.v.*) *transformation of one tissue into another*.

metastasis** (pl. **metastases**): (meta-***, *q.v.*, + G. ***stasis***, *state, condition, position*) *dispersion of cells* (generally diseased cells) *from one site to another via blood or lymph*.

microbe: (G. ***mikros***, *small*, + G. ***bios***, *life*) *a small living organism* (such as a **bacterium**).

morphogeny: (G. ***morph-***, *form, shape*, + G. ***gen-***, *origin* – cf. suffix ***-gen***) *development* (of structure).

morphology*: (G. ***morph-***, *form, shape*, + ***-logy***, *q.v.*) *the study or science of structure* (as opposed to function – cf. **physiology**).

myalgia*: (G. ***mus***, *muscle*, + G. ***algos***, *pain* + ***-ia***, *q.v.*) *muscle pain*.

myasthenia*: (G. ***mus***, *muscle*, + G. ***asthenēs***, *weak*, + ***-ia***, *q.v.*) *muscle weakness*.

myenteric: (G. ***mus***, *muscle*, + G. ***enteron***, *guts*) *related to intestinal muscle*.

myopathy*: (G. ***mus,*** *muscle,* + ***-pathy,*** *q.v.*) *disease of muscle.*

myopia*: (G. ***muōps,*** *short-sighted,* from ***muein,*** *to close, to be shut* (of the eyes), + ***ōps,*** *eye*; + ***-ia,*** *q.v.*) *shortsightedness* (in view of the existence of the term **hypermetropia,** *q.v.,* **hypometropia** would be a better term than **myopia**).

N

narcosis*: (G. ***narkē,*** *numbness,* + ***-osis,*** *q.v.*) *general* (as opposed to local) *anaesthesia.*

nausea: (L. noun meaning *sickness,* = G. ***nausia*** or ***nautia,*** *sea sickness,* from ***naus,*** *ship*) *the feeling which precedes and accompanies vomiting.*

necrosis*: (G. ***nekrōsis,*** *mortification*, from ***nekros,*** *corpse*) *death of a tissue or organ.*

neonatal: (G. ***neos,*** *new,* + L. ***natalis,*** *relating to birth*) *relating to the newborn.*

nephritis* (G. ***nephros,*** *kidney,* + ***-itis,*** *q.v.*) *inflammation of the kidney* (but the term has a special pathological significance not implied in the etymology).

neurectomy: (G. ***neuron,*** *sinew, tendon,* later *nerve,* + G. ***ektom-,*** *cutting out*) *removal of a nerve or part of a nerve.*

neurilemma: (G. ***neuron,*** *sinew, tendon,* later *nerve,* + G. ***lemma,*** *husk, rind*) *the outer covering of a nerve.*

neuroglia: (G. ***neuron,*** *sinew, tendon,* later *nerve,* + late and rare noun ***glia,*** *glue*) *supporting tissue of nerve cells in central nervous system.*

neurology*: (G. ***neuron,*** *sinew, tendon,* later *nerve,* + ***-logy,*** *q.v.*) *the study or science of nerves and the nervous system.*

neuropathy*: (G. ***neuron,*** *sinew, tendon,* later *nerve,* + ***-pathy,*** *q.v.*) *disease in nerves and the nervous system.*

nociceptor: (L. ***nocere,*** *to injure,* + L. ***-cept-***, from ***capere,*** *to take*) *receptor responding to injury* (cf. **exteroceptor**).

nulliparous: (L. ***nullus,*** *none,* + L. ***parere,*** *to bring forth, to bear*) *never having borne a child.*

O

obstetrics: (L. ***obstetrix***, *midwife*) *the study of pregnancy and the practice of midwifery.*

occlusion: (L. ***occludere/occlus-***, *to close, to shut up*)
1. *closure or blockage of conduction* (in a lymphatic or blood vessel, sometimes also in a nerve pathway).
2. *the relationship of the upper and lower teeth when the mouth is closed.*

odontoblast: (G. ***odous/odont-***, *tooth,* + G. ***blastos***, *shoot, germ*) *a tooth-forming* (specifically, dentine-forming) *cell* (cf. **osteoblast**).

oedema: (G. ***oidēma***, *a swelling*) *an accumulation of watery fluid* (not blood) *in the tissues* (frequently causing swelling) adj. **oedematous**).

-oid*: suffix derived from G. ***eidos***, *form,* and connoting *formed like.*

olfactory: (L. ***olfacere/olfact-***, *to smell* – active not passive) *related to the sense of smell.*

oligaemia*: (G. ***oligos***, *little, few,* + ***haem-***, *q.v.*, + ***-ia***, *q.v.*) *a reduced blood volume.*

-ology*: see **-logy***.

-oma*: suffix used in the formation of names of tumours or other morbid growths.

oncology*: (G. ***onkos***, *bulk, that which is distended,* + ***-logy***, *q.v.*) *the study or science of tumours.*

oogenesis*: (G. ***ōon***, *egg,* + ***-genesis***, *q.v.*) *egg development and production.*

ophthalmology*: (G. ***ophthalmos***, *eye,* + ***-logy***, *q.v.*) *the study or science of the eyes and vision.*

opisthotonos: (G. ***opisth-***, *behind, at the back,* + G. ***tonos***, *that which is stretched,* hence *strain, tension*) *contraction of the back muscles* (resulting in arching of the back).

***ortho-:** G. prefix meaning *upright, straight, correct.*

orthopaedic:** (ortho-***, *q.v.*, + G. ***pais/paid-*** (also diminutive form ***paidion***), *child*) *connected with the correction of deformities* (literally *in children,* but in people generally).

***orthostatic:** (**ortho-**, q.v., +G. **statos**, standing) related to the upright posture.*

-osis*: suffix found in a wide range of words, often indicating a pathological condition.

osteoblast: (G. ***osteon***, *bone,* +G. ***blastos***, *shoot, germ*) *a bone-forming cell.*

osteocyte*: (G. ***osteon***, *bone,* + ***-cyte***, *q.v.*) *a bone cell* (cf. **histiocyte**).

osteolysis*: (G. ***osteon***, *bone,* + ***-lysis***, *q.v.*) *bone absorption* (dissolution).

osteomalacia*: (G. ***osteon***, *bone,* + G. ***malakos***, *soft,* + ***ia***, *q.v.*) *softening of the bones.*

osteoporosis*: (G. ***osteon***, *bone,* +G. ***poros***, *passage through,* + ***-osis***, *q.v.*) *loss of calcified content of bone – rarefaction* (without change in shape).

otorhinolaryngology*: (G. ***ous/ōt-***, *ear,* +G. ***rhis/rhin-***, *nose,* +G. ***larunx/larung-***, *larynx,* + ***-logy***, *q.v.*) *the study or science of the ears, nose and throat.*

oxytocin: (G. ***oxus***, *sharp,* +G. ***tokos***, *childbirth*) *a hormone which speeds childbirth.*

P

paediatrics: (G. ***pais/paid-***, also diminutive form ***paidion***, *child,* +G. ***iatros***, *doctor, one who heals*) *the medical treatment of children.*

palaeocerebellum: (G. ***palaios***, *old, ancient,* +L. ***cerebellum***, *small brain,* diminutive of ***cerebrum***, *brain*) *the older part of the cerebellum, phylogenetically* (i.e. 'evolutionarily', – cf. **phylogeny**).

panacea: (G. ***panakeia***, *universal cure,* from G. ***pas/pan/pant-***, *all,* +G. ***akos***, *cure*) *a remedy for all diseases.*

pandemic: (G. ***pandēmos***, *spread throughout all the people, general,* from G. ***pas/pan/pant-***, *all*, + G. ***dēmos***, *people*) *a widespread disease.*

***para-:** G. prefix whose chief meanings in Eng. compounds are *by the side* and *amiss, wrong.*

paraesthesia*:** (para-***, *q.v.*, + ***aesthesia***, *q.v.*) *abnormal sensation* (cf. **an-** and **hyperaesthesia**).

parathyroid:** (para-***, *q.v.*, + G. ***thureos***, *an oblong shield* – ***thura***, the ultimate derivation, means *door* – whence *thyroid, shield-shaped*) *alongside, adjacent to, the thyroid gland.*

pathognomonic: (G. ***pathos***, *experience, that which one suffers*, + G. ***gnōmōn***, *a person who interprets or discerns*, also devices for doing the same, e.g. *pointer of sundial, carpenter's square*, etc.) *distinguishing feature or characteristic of a disease.*

pathology*: (G. ***pathos***, *experience, that which one suffers*, + ***-logy***, *q.v.*) *the study or science of disease.*

-pathy*: suffix which in Eng. compounds often connotes *disease*, from G. ***pathos***, *experience, feeling*, i.e. *that which happens to one*, or *that which one suffers.*

***peri-:** G. prefix meaning *around.*

pericardium:** (peri-***, *q.v.*, + G. ***kardia***, *heart*) *that* (membranous sac) *which surrounds the heart.*

periodontoclasia*:** (peri-***, *q.v.*, + G. ***odous/odont-***, *tooth*, + G. ***klasis***, *breaking*, from ***klaein***, *to break*, + ***-ia***, *q.v.*) *degeneration or destruction of the tissues surrounding the tooth.*

peristalsis:** (peri-***, *q.v.*, + G. ***stalsis***, *checking*, i.e. *compressing*) literally *contractions around* (applied to waves of contraction and relaxation which pass along the gut).

perivascular:** (peri-***, *q.v.*, + L. ***vasculum***, *small vessel*, diminutive of ***vas***, *vessel*) *around a vessel.*

phaeochromocyte* (G. ***phaios***, *grey, darkish*, + G. ***chrōma***, *colour*, + ***cyte***, *q.v.*) *dark staining* (with chromic salts) *cell* (found in the sympathetic ganglia and suprarenal glands).

phagocyte*: (G. ***phagein***, *to eat*, + ***-cyte***, *q.v.*) *a cell capable of* *ingesting and digesting other cells* (including micro-organisms).

pharmacology*: (G. ***pharmakon***, *a drug*, + ***-logy***, *q.v.*) *the study or science of drugs.*

phonation: (G. ***phōnē***, *voice*) *the production of sounds used in speech.*

phylogeny: (G. ***phulon***, *trace, tribe* + ***gen-***, *origin* – cf. suffix ***-gen***) *the development* or *the evolution of a species.*

physiology*: (G. ***phusis***, *natural growth*, + ***-logy***, *q.v.*) *the study or science of functions* (as opposed to structures) *in living things (cf.* **morphology**).

placebo: (L. verb-form meaning *I shall please*) *a medicine or a form of treatment given to please or reassure a patient* (a substance which has no pharmacological action).

plethysmograph: (G. ***plēthuein***, *to swell*, + ***-graph***, see **angiocardiogram**) *an apparatus for recording volume change.*

pneumonia*: (G. ***pneumōn*** (or ***pleumōn***), *lung*, + ***-ia***, *q.v.*) *inflammation of the lung.*

poikilothermal: (G. ***poikilos***, *speckled, variegated*, + G. ***thermos***, *hot*) *variable temperature* (usually that of the environment) applied to cold-blooded animals (cf. **homoeothermal**).

polymorphic: (G. ***polus***, *many*, + G. ***morph-***, *form, shape*) *having many shapes* (applied to a class of white corpuscles of which the nucleus has many shapes – often called 'polymorphonuclear').

***post-:** L. prefix meaning *behind* or *after.*

postnatal:** (post-***, *q.v.*, + L. ***natalis***, *relating to birth*) *after birth.*

post-ocular:** (post-***, *q.v.*, + L. ***oculus***, *eye*) *behind the eye.*

***pre-:** L. prefix meaning *before, in front of.*

precordium:** (pre-***, *q.v.*, + L. ***cor/cordis***, *heart*) *the region in front of the heart* (and stomach).

presbyopia*: (G. ***presbus***, *an old man*, + G. ***ōps***, *eye*, + ***-ia***, *q.v.*) *impaired vision in old age.*

***pro-:** G. prefix meaning *beforehand.*

proctalgia*: (G. ***prōktos***, *anus,* + G. **algos**, *pain,* + **-ia**, *q.v.*) *pain in the anus or rectum.*

prognosis:** (pro-***, *q.v.,* + G. ***gnōsis***, *knowledge*) *forecast* (of the course of a disease).

prophylaxis:** (pro-***, *q.v.,* + G. ***phulassein/phulax-***, *guard against*) *disease prevention.*

proprioceptor: (L. ***proprius***, *one's own,* + ***-cept-***, from ***capere***, *to take*) *receptor which responds to stimuli originating within an organism itself* (cf. **exteroceptor** and **nociceptor**).

prosencephalon: (G. ***prosō***, *forwards,* + G. ***enkephalon***, *the brain*) *the forebrain.*

prosthesis: (G. noun meaning *addition, attachment*) *an artificial replacement for a limb or other part of the body.*

protein: (G. ***prōtos***, *first, chief in importance*) originally *the most important constituents of the body* (reserved for a class of biochemical compounds with large molecules and containing nitrogen).

psychiatry: (G. ***psuchē***, a notoriously complex word meaning *soul, life, spirit, breath,* + G. ***iatros***, *doctor, one who heals*) *the treatment of the mind.*

ptyalin: (G. ***ptualon***, *saliva*) a term formerly used for *the digestive enzyme in saliva* (current term is **amylase**, *q.v.*).

puerperal: (L. ***puerperium***, *childbirth*) *relating to childbirth.*

pyrexia*: (G. ***puretos***, *fever,* from ***pur***, *fire,* + **-ia**, *q.v.*) *high body-temperature; fever.*

R

radiograph: (L. ***radius***, *beam, ray,* + ***-graph***, see **angiocardiogram**) *a tracing* (photograph) *obtained with X-rays.*

radiotherapy: (L. ***radius***, *beam, ray,* + G. ***therapeia***, *care, treatment*) *treatment using radiation.*

refractory: (rare L. word ***refractarius***, *stubborn*) *unresponsive or resistant* (to stimulation or treatment).

reticular: (L. ***reticulum***, *a little net*) *net-like in appearance.*

***retro-:** L. prefix meaning *backwards.*

retroflexion:** (retro-***, *q.v.*, + L. ***flectere/flex-***, *to bend*) *being bent backwards.*

rhinology*: (G. ***rhis/rhin-***, *nose,* + ***-logy***, *q.v.*) *the study or science of the nose.*

rostral: (L. ***rostrum***, *snout, beak*) *relating to upper end of the body.*

S

sarcolemma: (G. ***sarx/sark-***, *flesh,* + G. ***lemma***, *husk, rind*) *the membrane covering muscle fibres* (**myolemma** would be a better word).

schizophrenia*: (G. ***schizein***, *to split,* + G. ***phren-***, *mind* – literally, *diaphragm,* or *midriff*, but regarded by Greeks as a location of what we call *mental activity,* + ***-ia***, *q.v.*) *split mind* (a mental disorder with characteristic signs and symptoms).

seminiferous: (L. ***semen/seminis***, *seed,* + L. ***ferre***, *to bear*) *carrying semen.*

sialagogue: (G. ***sialon***, *saliva,* + G. ***agōgos***, *leading*) *a substance which excites salivary flow.*

somaesthesia*: (G. ***sōma***, *body,* + ***aesthesia***, *q.v.*) *sensation depending on receptors widely distributed throughout the body.*

sphygmograph: (G. ***sphugmos***, *beating, pulsation,* + ***-graph***, see **angiocardiogram**) *a device for recording the pulse.*

splanchnic: (G. ***splanchna***, *the inward parts*) *relating to the abdominal organs*

stereognosis: (G. ***stereos***, *firm, solid,* + G. ***gnōsis***, *knowledge*) *knowledge of the size and shape of objects* (obtained by touching them).

stomatology*: (G. ***stoma/stomatos***, *mouth,* + ***-logy***, *q.v.*) *the study or science of the mouth.*

streptococcus (pl. **-cocci**): (G. ***streptos***, *pliant, easily twisted,* + G. ***kokkos***, *grain, seed, berry*) *oval or round microorganisms seen in twisted chains.*

stroma (pl. **stromata**): (G. ***strōma***, *bed or mattress*) *the supporting framework of a cell or organ.*

***sub-:** L. prefix meaning *under,* or *moderately, partially, incompletely.*

subcranial:** (sub-***, *q.v.*, + G. **kranion**, skull) *beneath the skull.*

***supra-:** L. prefix meaning *above.*

suprarenal:** (supra-***, *q.v.*, + L. **renes**, *kidneys*) *above the kidneys* (suprarenal glands lie just above the kidneys).

***sym-/syn-:** G. prefix connoting *with, together.*

symphysis:** (sym-***, *q.v.*, + G. ***phusis***, *natural growth*) *a growing-together or union* (e.g. of two bones).

symptom: (G. ***sumptōma***, *an occurrence, an attribute*, esp. *a symptom*) *a feature of a disease experienced by the patient,* e.g. giddiness (as opposed to a sign, which is what an observer sees or records – e.g. spots).

syncytium** (pl. **-cytia**): (sym-/syn-***, *q.v.*, + ***cyt-***, *see* ***-cyte***) *a mass of cells, interconnected in some way.*

synergist:** (sym-/syn-***, *q.v.*, + G. **ergon**, *work, function*) *an agent* (muscle or drug) *which acts with another.*

T

tachycardia*: (G. ***tachus***, swift, + G. ***kardia***, *heart*, + ***-ia***, *q.v.*) *rapid heart rate.*

telencephalon: (G. ***telos***, *end*, + G. **enkephalon**, *brain*) *the hindbrain* (cf. **prosencephalon**).

topography: (G. ***topos***, *place*, + G. ***graphein***, *to write*) *study of the position of parts of the body.*

toxicology*: (G. ***toxikos***, see **toxin**, + ***-logy***, *q.v.*) *the study or science of poisons.*

toxin: (G. ***toxikos***, *connected with a bow and arrow,* then, when applied to a drug, *for smearing arrows with* – hence, by implication, *poisonous*) *a poisonous substance.*

***trans-:** L. prefix meaning *across*.

transfusion:** (trans-***, *q.v.*, + L. ***fundere/fus-***, *to pour*) *process of conveying a fluid* (from one vessel to another).

traumatic: (G. ***trauma/traumat-***, *a wound*) *relating to injury*.

V

vasoconstrictor: (L. ***vas***, *vessel*, + L. ***constringere/constrict-***, *to tie together*) *causing* (blood-)*vessel constriction*.

ventroflexion: (L. ***venter/ventris***, *belly*, + L. ***flectere/flex-***, *to bend*) *bending forwards*.

X

xerostomia*: (G. ***xeros***, *dry*, + G. ***stoma***, *mouth*, + ***-ia***, *q.v.*) *dryness of the mouth*.